For information contact:

MBS Publishing LLC
Atlanta, Georgia 30031, USA
www.microgreensworld.com

Pamphlet and Cover design by Andrew Neves
Photos by Twenty20

First Edition: April 2020

10 9 8 7 6 5 4 3 2 1

To Geb, Auset, and Het-Heru; to T and my sons; and my dear friends G-Man and Jonesy.

CONTENTS

ENDORSEMENTS

"Very Informative. This will definitely open your eyes and get you eating much better for your health." – *Jennifer Willison*

"What we eat matters. This read opened my eyes. Enlightened me on the power of micro greens. Clearly well researched." – *Liz*

"Useful and delicious. This book provides useful and delicious recipes for everyday green menus. Recommended."

Jennifer Xue *is an award-winning, multi-book author and syndicated columnist based in Northern California.*

WANT MORE FREE BOOKS?

Andrew Neves is giving away a free starter library

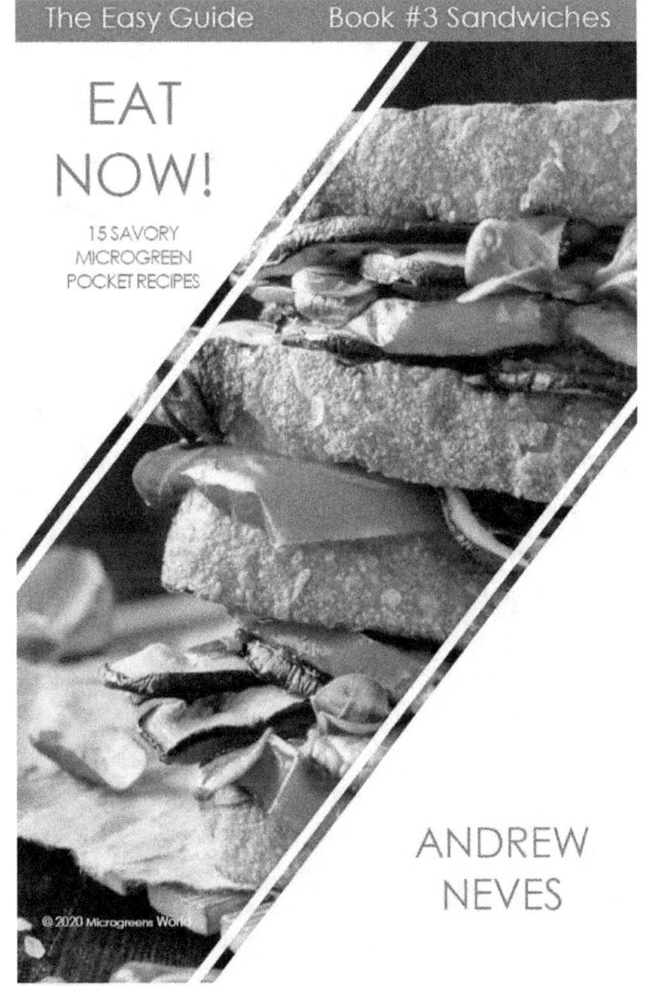

If you like **FREE**, then <u>**CLICK HERE FOR YOUR FREE BOOKS**</u>

Microgreens World

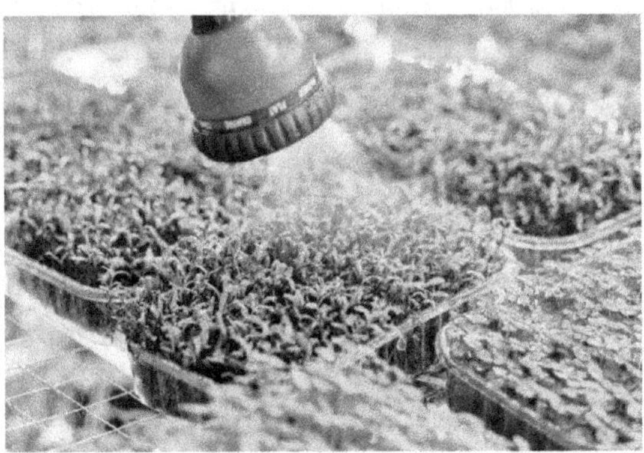

You're in the right place.

Get the most up-to-date information about microgreens from across the world.

Nutrition | Science | Trends
© 2019 Microgreens World

Visit Microgreens World: www.microgreensworld.com

This cookbook is lighthearted and devoted to people who delight in tasty and nutritious food.

Microgreens are becoming the rage as more people learn how easy it is to grow, prepare, and eat.

I took the soup recipes in this pocket cookbook from cultures in the Western Hemisphere (North America, Central and South America, and the Caribbean).

You should adapt the soup dishes to make use of the foods that grow in your own community.

Now, what if I told you that each recipe comes with Nutrition Facts, including calorie count, vitamins, and minerals?

These are light soup recipes with as little as 80 calories each. You can have a bowl of soup at lunch or a cup of soup as an addition to your evening meal.

Read through the nutrition labels for a snapshot of each recipe's nutritional profile.

If the label lists less than 5 percent daily value for a nutrient, it is low, while 20 percent or more is high.

You want to limit saturated fat, cholesterol, and sodium, and get enough fiber, vitamins, and minerals.

This pocket cookbook is also a handy guide to plan quick meals for those days when you're in a hurry.

You can find many of the ingredients at your local farmers' markets and supermarkets.

You can order other ingredients online and have them shipped directly to your door in a matter of hours or days.

For those of you who are new to microgreens, may this book encourage a new and happy familiarity with food that you can grow yourself.

Sincerely,

THE GREAT DEBATE: TO HEAT OR NOT TO HEAT MICROGREENS

So, we know a few things about mighty microgreens.

- Research in the past five years has tripled.
- Demand is increasing, and supermarkets and food establishments are making them available locally.
- There is no question that they are the "latest thing" in the culinary world.

Microgreens have become popular in North America, North Europe, Asia, and Oceania.

And more and more chefs, are preparing more and more dishes, that cater to more and more health-conscious consumers like you who are particularly attentive to your health, diet, and food quality.

But these same chefs are still only using microgreens to "enhance" salads or as edible garnishes to embellish a wide variety of other dishes.

And if you scour the Internet, but for the infrequent exception, everybody discourages "cooking" microgreens because they say you lose nutritional value.

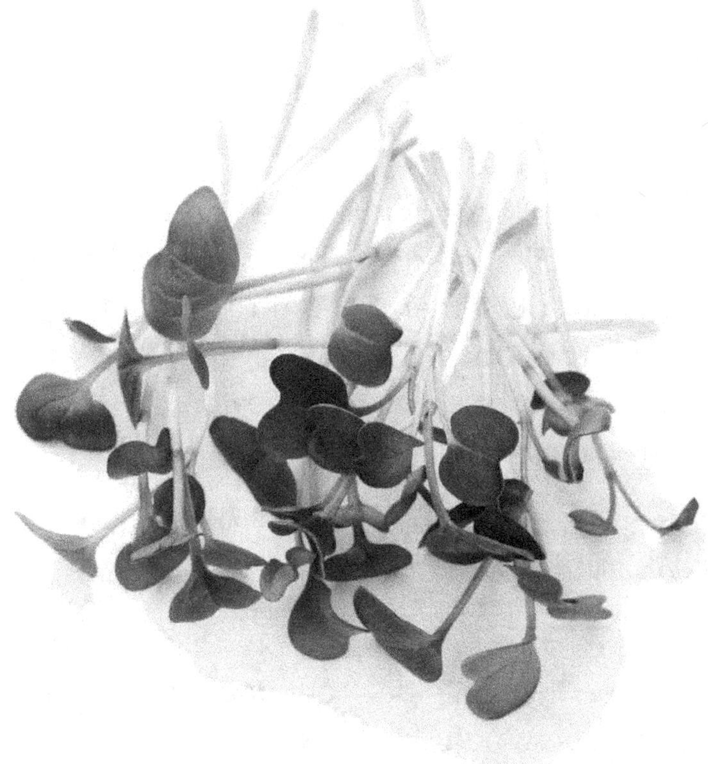

But no one seems to have quantified just "how much nutritional value do you lose?"

So, I set out to find out, because I wanted your 15 Microgreen Soup Recipes to be indeed savory and tasty.

What the Science Says

An <u>International Journal of Scientific and Technology Research study</u> looked at the effects of heat on different vegetables. It measured the percentage of vitamin C lost at 5, 15, and 30 minutes while exposed to a constant temperature of 140°F (60°C).

The pain threshold for your tongue is about 153°F (67.2°C)[PDF]).

Vegetable Samples	% Lost in 5 min	%lost in 15 min	%lost in 30 min
Pepper	11.76	35.28	64.71
Green Pea	10.59	33.33	58.28
Spinach	9.94	29.94	60.00
Pumpkin	12.43	37.43	62.43
Carrot	16.57	33.33	49.91
Average Loss	12.26	33.86	59.07

Table 1. % loss in concentration of Vitamin C as heating time varies

The most thermolabile (*definition: readily destroyed or deactivated by heat*) of vitamins is folate (vitamin B9), followed by vitamin B1 (thiamin), B6 (pyridoxine), and vitamin C. Still, most vitamins are thermolabile to some extent.

As the authors state: "Vitamin C is water-soluble [more on this later] and, as such, is easily leached into the water and then degraded by heat."

But what does that mean for you and me?

Getting Your Recommended Daily Allowance (RDA)

If you are an <u>adult of medium weight</u>, eating about 41g (1.45 oz) of **red cabbage microgreens** is enough for your RDA (*see more later*) of Vitamin C (60mg).

Region	Adult population	Average weight
Latin America | Caribbean	386M	67.9 kg (149.7 lb)
North America	263M	80.7 kg (177.9 lb)
Oceania	24M	74.1 kg (163.4 lb)
World	4,630M	62.0 kg (136.7 lb)

Table 2: Source, Wikipedia, <u>Human Body Weight</u>

And, 15g (0.53 oz) of green radish microgreens would satisfy the RDA of Vitamin E (13mg). Just 17g (0.46 oz) of garnet amaranth microgreens would be enough to fulfill the RDA of Vitamin K (70ug).

What We Know That Works

Now, when compared to similar conventional vegetables often used to cook, the consumption of raw microgreens has three times more nutrients.

"Cooking" these same microgreens for 5 minutes in 140-180°F soup pot will still yield you at least 80-85% of the nutrient value.

That is 200% more than cooked green vegetables!

Microgreens are a rich food source for a demanding consumer like you.

Someone who can diversify and enrich your diet using a large variety of available microgreens.

All 15 of your recipes call for 5 minutes of "cooking."

So, enjoy them!

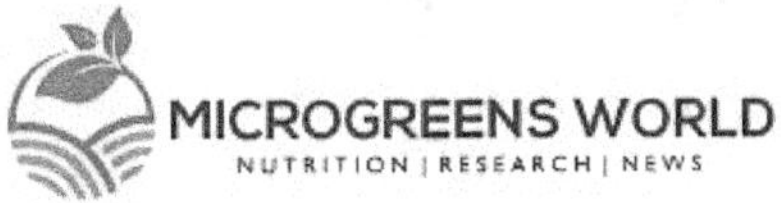

Visit Microgreens World: http://microgreensworld.com/

BARBADOS SALT-FREE CARROT MICROGREENS VEGETABLE SOUP

Carrot microgreens taste like carrot roots and are a superbly rich source of antioxidants, carotenes and vitamin A.

Microgreen	Taste	Aroma	Flavor	Intensity
Carrot	Sweet		Crunchy	Mild

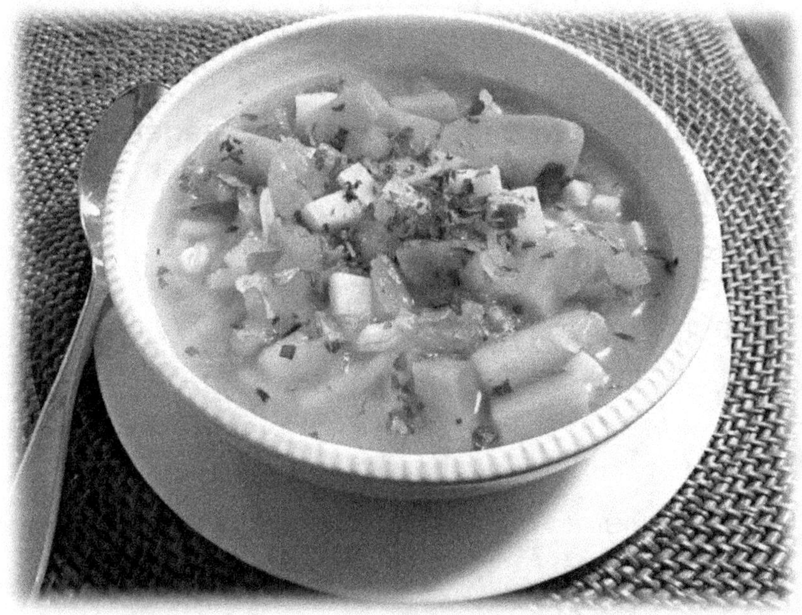

This is a substantial soup that will satisfy the largest of appetites. A real salt-free feast that requires only fresh fruit juice to complete the meal.

Barbados Salt-Free Carrot Microgreens Vegetable Soup

Prep Time	40 mins

Course: Soup

Cuisine: Caribbean

Keyword: carrot microgreens

Servings: 4-6 people   Calories: 323 kcal

Equipment

- 4-Quart Soup pot or saucepan

Ingredients

- 4 cups carrot microgreens
- 1 lb (450 g) yam
- 1/2 lb (225 g) sweet potato
- 1 lb (450 g) pumpkin
- 1 lb (450 g) callaloo (or spinach)
- 1/2 small cabbage
- 1/2 lb (225 g) carrots
- 1 chayote
- 1 green pepper
- 2 cloves garlic
- 2 medium-sized tomatoes
- 3 spring onions
- 2 pts (1100 ml) water

Instructions

1. First, prepare the vegetables.
2. Peel the yam, sweet potato, and pumpkin and cut into large cubes, removing the seeds from the pumpkin.
3. Carefully wash the callaloo, trimming away any thick stems and chop.
4. Coarsely chop the cabbage, being careful to discard the outer leaves, peel and slice the carrots.
5. Peel the chayote, cut it lengthways into quarters, and remove the heart.
6. Roughly dice the chayote and green pepper, peel and chop the tomatoes and slice the spring onions.
7. Place the pumpkin and root vegetables in a large saucepan with the water.
8. Bring to the boil and simmer for 10 minutes.
9. Add to the pan the callaloo, cabbage, chayote, pepper, and finally, the chopped tomatoes and spring onions.
10. Season with plenty of freshly ground black pepper and simmer for 15 minutes more until cooked.
11. Add the microgreens and cook for 5 minutes more.
12. Serve warm.

Nutrition Facts

Serving size: 2 cups

Servings: 4

Amount per serving

Calories 323

% Daily Value*

Total Fat 1g	**1%**
Saturated Fat 0.3g	**1%**
Cholesterol 0mg	**0%**
Sodium 472mg	**21%**
Total Carbohydrate 75g	**27%**
Dietary Fiber 17.9g	**64%**
Total Sugars 19.6g	
Protein 8.3g	
Vitamin D 0mcg	0%
Calcium 161mg	12%
Iron 6mg	34%
Potassium 1920mg	41%

*The % Daily Value (DV) tells you how much a nutrient in a food serving contributes to a daily diet. 2,000 calorie a day is used for general nutrition advice.

Recipe analyzed by very**well**

HAWAIIAN CREAMED BREADFRUIT SOUP WITH SUNFLOWER MICROGREENS

A traditional staple in Hawaii and the Caribbean, and rich in phytonutrients, breadfruit is sometimes called the tree potato, for its potato-like consistency when cooked.

Microgreen	Taste	Aroma	Flavor	Intensity
Sunflower	Sweet		Nutty	Mild

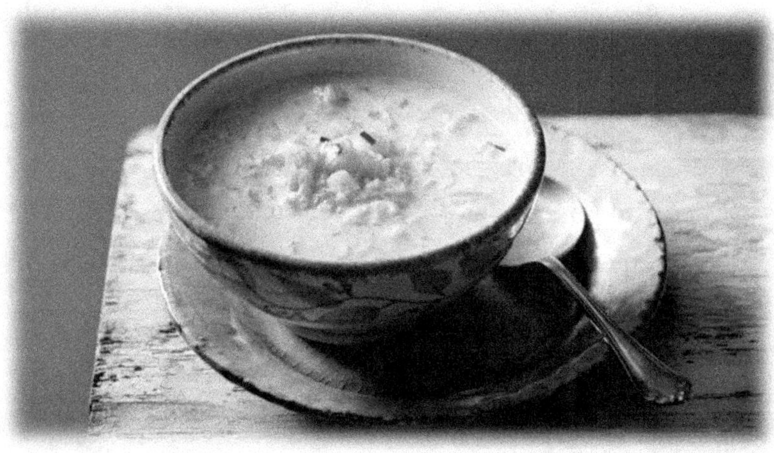

Breadfruit tastes a bit like artichoke, and when paired with the nutty flavor of sunflower microgreens, this soup makes for a delicious and creamy meal.

Hawaiian Cream of Breadfruit Soup with Sunflower Microgreens

11

Prep Time	35 mins

Course: Soup

Cuisine: Hawaiian

Keyword: sunflower microgreens

Servings: 4 people

Calories: 175 kcal

Equipment

- Large saucepan; blender.

Ingredients

- ½ cup sunflower microgreens
- 2 medium-sized onions
- 2 cloves garlic
- ½ lb. (225 g) (fresh | canned breadfruit)
- 2 tbsp sunflower oil
- 1 bay leaf
- 1½ pint vegetable stock
- ½ pint (300 ml) low-fat milk
- 1 tbsp spring onion tops
- ½ tsp ground black pepper to taste

Instructions

1. Peel the garlic cloves and chop finely.
2. Open the breadfruit can and pour off the brine.
3. Remove the breadfruit and dice.
4. Heat the vegetable oil in a large saucepan.
5. Sauté the onion and garlic until soft, but not colored.
6. Add the diced breadfruit, bay leaf, and vegetable stock.
7. Bring to a boil, cover pan, and simmer on low heat until the breadfruit is tender.
8. Remove the bay leaf and liquidize the soup in the blender.
9. Return the soup to the saucepan, add microgreens, milk, and black pepper.
10. Reheat gently, taking care not to boil.
11. Serve sprinkled with chopped onion tops

Note: If you're unable to find fresh breadfruit, canned, ripe breadfruit is a good substitute.

Nutrition Facts

Serving size: cups

Servings: 4

Amount per serving

Calories 180

% Daily Value*

Total Fat 10.8g	14%
Saturated Fat 1.3g	7%
Cholesterol 3mg	1%
Sodium 99mg	4%
Total Carbohydrate 18g	7%
Dietary Fiber 3.7g	13%
Total Sugars 9.3g	
Protein 4.8g	
Vitamin D 32mcg	159%
Calcium 100mg	8%
Iron 1mg	4%
Potassium 341mg	7%

*The % Daily Value (DV) tells you how much a nutrient in a food serving contributes to a daily diet. 2,000 calorie a day is used for general nutrition advice.

Recipe analyzed by very**well**

JAMAICAN CURRIED LENTIL AND RADISH MICROGREENS SOUP WITH COCONUT

Radish microgreens have a sweet flavor. Some varieties are as hot and pungent as a mature radish root.

Microgreen	Taste	Aroma	Flavor	Intensity
Radish	Sweet			Strong

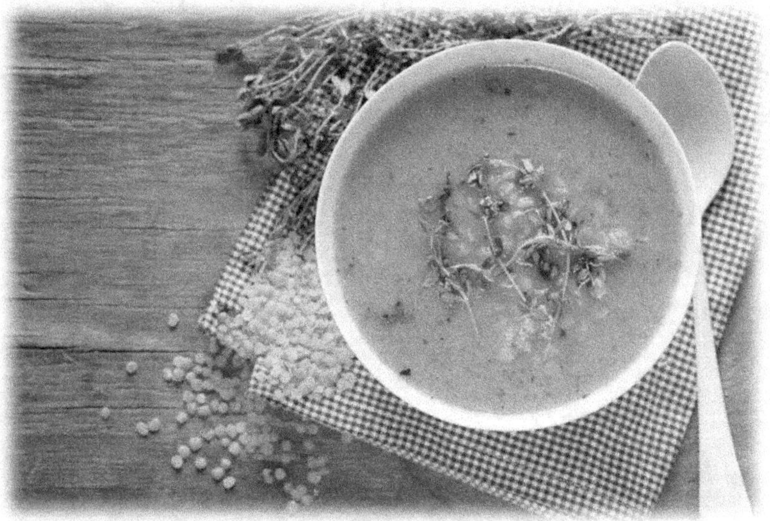

This curry lentil soup is easy to cook and great as a main dish for vegetarians and non-vegetarians. Add with the sweet flavor of radish, coconut, and ginger, and it is your tasty lunch-time favorite.

Jamaican Curried Lentil and Radish Microgreens Soup with Coconut

Prep Time	60 mins

Course:	Cuisine:	Keyword:
Soup	Caribbean	radish microgreens

Servings: 4 people   Calories: 420 kcal

Equipment

- Pestle and mortar. Saucepan or soup pot (6-quart)

Ingredients

- 2 oz radish microgreens
- 1 medium-sized onion
- 2 cloves garlic
- 2 slices peeled root ginger
- 1 small red pepper
- 1 small green pepper
- 2 tbs vegetable oil
- 2 tsp ground coriander
- 1 tsp ground cumin
- 1 tsp garam masala
- 2 oz (55g) creamed coconut
- 1¾ pint (1 liter) vegetable stock
- 4 oz (115 g) split red lentils
- 1 scotch bonnet pepper
- * freshly ground black pepper to taste

Instructions

1. Peel and chop the onion.
2. Crush the peeled cloves of garlic and the slices of ginger together using a pestle and mortar, adding a little water to produce a thick paste.
3. Slice the red and green peppers into strips.
4. Heat the vegetable oil in a large saucepan, add the chopped onion and fry on medium heat until transparent.
5. Add the garlic and ginger paste and cook for two minutes before putting in the spices.
6. Fry the spices for another minute then stir in the red and green peppers.
7. Roughly grate the creamed coconut into the pan and stir until it has blended to make a thick sauce.
8. Add the vegetable stock, the washed lentils, the whole hot pepper, and black pepper.
9. Simmer the soup for 30 minutes.
10. Add microgreens and cook for 5-10 more minutes
11. Stir occasionally being careful not to crush the hot pepper.
12. Remove the hot pepper before serving

Nutrition Facts

Serving size: 2 cups

Servings: 4

Amount per serving

Calories 420

% Daily Value*

Total Fat 16.9g	**22%**
Saturated Fat 9.1g	**46%**
Cholesterol 0mg	**0%**
Sodium 4491mg	**195%**
Total Carbohydrate 53.3g	**19%**
Dietary Fiber 19g	**68%**
Total Sugars 21.3g	
Protein 9.6g	
Vitamin D 0mcg	0%
Calcium 207mg	16%
Iron 6mg	34%
Potassium 479mg	10%

*The % Daily Value (DV) tells you how much a nutrient in a food serving contributes to a daily diet. 2,000 calorie a day is used for general nutrition advice.

Recipe analyzed by very**well**

SOUTHWESTERN CHILLED CILANTRO AVOCADO SOUP

Cilantro microgreens are ideal when preparing most Southwestern United States and Asian dishes. They are deliciously intense and 8 ounces (1cup) contains about 5 calories, vitamins A, C, E and K, minerals and lutein.

Microgreen	Taste	Aroma	Flavor	Intensity
Cilantro	Lemony	Pungent	Citrus	Strong

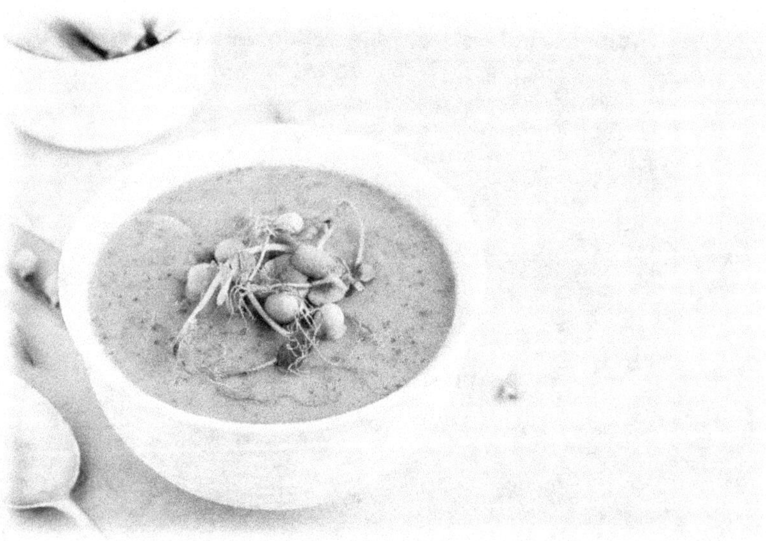

A beautiful green soup which is served refreshingly chilled on a warm spring day.

Southwestern Chilled Cilantro Avocado Soup

Prep Time	10 mins

Course: Soup

Cuisine: Southwestern USA

Keyword: cilantro microgreens

Servings: 4 people   Calories: 599 kcal

Equipment

- Blender

Ingredients

- 4 oz Cilantro microgreens   Rinsed and dried
- 3 Avocados (ripe)
- ½ Lime juiced | 1 tsp lime
- 1½ pint (850 ml) low-fat milk
- ½ tsp ground black pepper to taste

Instructions

1. Chop the cilantro microgreens.
2. Halve the avocados, remove the seed, and scoop the flesh.
3. Mash the avocados with the lime juice to make a puree.
4. Transfer to an electric blender
5. Blend the avocado, gradually pouring in the milk.
6. Stir in the chopped microgreens
7. Blend until thoroughly liquidized.
8. Season with the black pepper
9. Chill until ready to serve.

Nutrition Facts

Servings: 4

Amount per serving

Calories 599

% Daily Value*

Total Fat 36.1g	**46%**
Saturated Fat 10.4g	**52%**
Cholesterol 34mg	**11%**
Sodium 318mg	**14%**
Total Carbohydrate 48.5g	**18%**
Dietary Fiber 11.2g	**40%**
Total Sugars 36g	
Protein 26.2g	
Vitamin D 349mcg	1745%
Calcium 839mg	65%
Iron 2mg	10%
Potassium 1897mg	40%

*The % Daily Value (DV) tells you how much a nutrient in a food serving contributes to a daily diet. 2,000 calorie a day is used for general nutrition advice.

Recipe analyzed by very**well**

EAT TO MEET YOUR RDA: THE 12 MICROGREEN VITAMINS YOU NEED

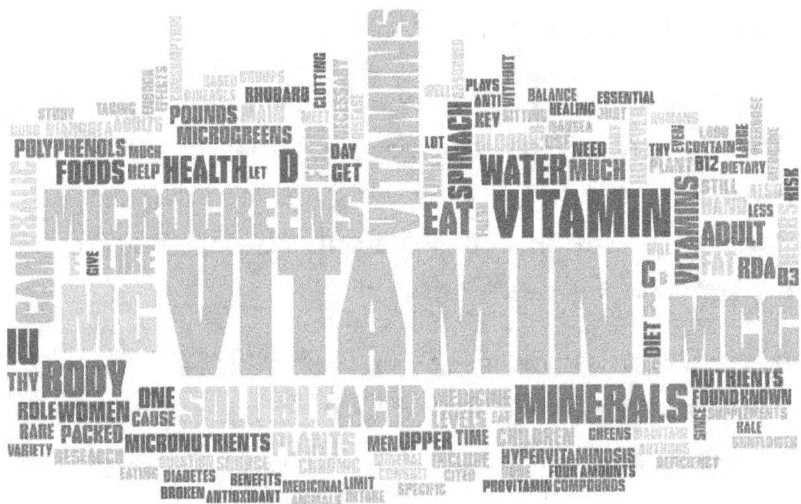

I've been sharing my microgreens growing with my neighbor Marty, and yesterday we were sitting on my deck when he asked me, **"about how much microgreens should you eat per day?"** That's an excellent question, I thought.

You should eat just enough microgreens to help you meet the <u>Recommended Dietary Allowance (RDA)</u> necessary to fulfill your nutritional requirements.

Tasty foods can make you overeat. So, you should be aware that some vitamins and minerals have a maximum daily dose to prevent adverse effects like nausea and diarrhea.

On the other hand, if you were lacking in some minerals or vitamins, you could choose to eat more microgreens to help close the gap. But, always consult your medical professionals before taking any herbs or supplements.

This recipe book will try to give you detailed answers to the question of how much microgreens you need and how **soups** are a great way to eat them.

Quick Reads

- <u>Let Microgreens Be Thy Medicine</u>
- <u>How Much More?</u>
- <u>Fat-soluble Vitamins Won't Make You Fat</u>
- <u>Water-soluble Vitamins Don't Stay</u>
- <u>When to Be Cautious</u>
- <u>Microgreens and Bad Body Odor</u>
- <u>Which Ones Should I Eat?</u>
- <u>Eat To Meet Your RDA</u>

Let Microgreens Be Thy Medicine

Plants have been the source of healing for thousands of years. Herbal medicine, the study and use of medicinal plants, is still widely practiced even in countries like the US and the UK.

Hippocrates, the 4th century B.C. Greek father of medicine, once said, "Let thy food be thy medicine and thy medicine be thy food." When it comes to chronic illnesses such as heart disease and diabetes, there is a lot of evidence that food has healing properties that can restore or maintain good health.

Microgreens are usually classified with seaweed, nutrition yeast, juicing grasses like wheatgrass, and herbs as "medicinal foods."

They have been cited as providing specific, measurable benefits, just like those of synthetic drugs.

And if you think about it, you use herbs like ginger, curry (curcumin), garlic, and basil all the time when you're cooking. And we know from research that like fresh herbs, microgreens contain large amounts of vitamins A, C, and K, as well as polyphenols.

Polyphenols are micronutrients exclusive to plants that have both antioxidant and anti-inflammatory capabilities.

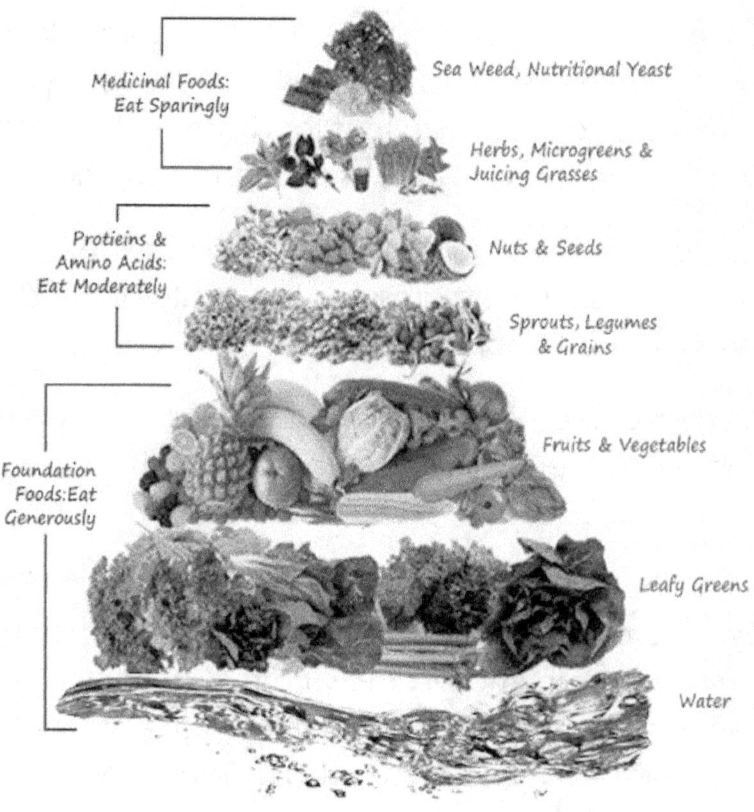

Figure 1. The Living Food Pyramid

In a 2009 study in the <u>Journal of Oxidative Medicine and Cellular Longevity</u>, the authors cited that "long term consumption of diets rich in plant polyphenols offer protection against the development of cancers, cardiovascular diseases, diabetes, osteoporosis, and neurodegenerative diseases."

The authors went on to show that polyphenols in herbs and other plant-based foods can also reduce chronic inflammation and its associated risk for chronic disease.

And while there is still a lot of research on microgreens to be done, eating more can always give you the health benefits. So, add more fresh microgreens to your diet!

How Much More?

You would have to eat 20-plus pounds of microgreens a day for a week to reach levels that could cause you any potential life-threatening harm.

According to the latest <u>National Poison Data System Annual Report</u>, vitamin overdose represented less than one quarter of 1% of all substance categories most frequently identified in calls.

Dietary supplements (including minerals) were even less than that, one-tenth of 1%.

Micronutrients, which include vitamins and minerals, are one of the major groups of nutrients your body needs.

Vitamins help key body processes like energy production, immune function, and blood clotting. Meanwhile, minerals are essential for processes like growth, bone health, and fluid balance.

Macronutrients, on the other hand, include proteins, fats, and carbohydrates.

Humans must obtain micronutrients from food since your body cannot produce vitamins and minerals — for the most part. That's why they're also referred to as essential nutrients.

Vitamins are organic compounds made by plants and animals, which can be broken down by heat, acid, or air. On the other hand, minerals are inorganic, exist in soil or water, and cannot be broken down.

When you eat, you consume the vitamins that plants and animals created or the minerals they absorbed.

The micronutrient content of each food microgreen is different, so it's best to eat a variety of foods to get enough vitamins and minerals.

An adequate intake of all micronutrients is necessary for optimal health, as each vitamin and mineral have a specific role in your body.

Vitamins and minerals are divided into four groups:

- water-soluble vitamins,
- fat-soluble vitamins,
- macro minerals, and
- trace minerals.

No matter what type, they are absorbed the same way in your body and work together in the body.

Vitamins are grouped based either as water-soluble or fat-soluble. Most vitamins are water-soluble. When you eat more than your body can use, they get flushed out in your pee. Fat-soluble vitamins, on the other hand, are like oils and don't dissolve in water.

Fat-soluble Vitamins Won't Make You Fat
There are four fat-soluble vitamins in the human diet.

Vitamin A helps maintain your vision. So much so that without it you would go blind. The primary sources of Vitamin A are retinoids and carotenoid antioxidants known as provitamin A.

The most efficient of these is beta-carotene, which is abundant in many microgreens, such as kale and spinach.

Upper Limit	Adult Men	Adult Women	Children
10,000 IU (900 mcg)	3,000 IU (900 mcg)	2,333 (700 mcg)	1,000 IU (300 mcg) to 2,000 IU (600 mcg)

Table 3. RDA for Vitamin A

Overdosing on vitamin A leads to an adverse condition known as hypervitaminosis A. Eating a lot of provitamin A does not cause hypervitaminosis, a very rare but a serious issue.

Vitamin D maintains the balance of calcium and phosphorus levels in your blood to maintain bone health.

The primary source of vitamin D is Vitamin D2, found in mushrooms and plants.

Amaranth and sunflower microgreens are packed with Vitamin D.

Upper Limit	Adults and Children	Elderly Adults
4,000 IU (100 mcg)	600 IU (15 mcg)	800 IU (20 mcg)

Table 4. RDA for Vitamin D

The vital signs of vitamin D deficiency include fatigue, weak muscles, soft bones, an increased risk of fractures, and susceptibility to infections.

Vitamin D overdoes, hypervitaminosis D, is extremely rare. It occurs if you take large amounts over time since extra vitamin D can build up in the body.

Vitamin E is a group of related antioxidant compounds (tocopherol and tocotrienol) which act in the body to protect cells against free radicals and oxidative damage.

Spinach, cilantro, green daikon radish, and sunflower microgreens are packed with Vitamin E.

Upper Limit	Adults and Children over 14	Breastfeeding Women
1500 IU (1,000 mg)	22 IU (15 mg/s) of alpha tocopherol	28 IU (19 mg)

Table 5. RDA for Vitamin E

Vitamin E deficiency is rare in humans. Like all fat-soluble vitamins, vitamin E can accumulate to toxic levels over time, so it's possible to overdose on this vitamin.

Vitamin K plays a crucial role in blood clotting. Without it, you would run the risk of bleeding to death. The primary dietary forms are vitamin K1, found in plant foods.

Spinach, kale, and broccoli microgreens are packed with Vitamin K.

However, consult your physician as Vitamin K can affect the liver, and should never be taken as a supplement if a patient is on blood thinners,

Upper Limit	Adult Men	Adult Women	Children
UNKNOWN	120 mcg	90 mcg	30-75 mcg

Table 6. RDA for Vitamin k

Water-soluble Vitamins Don't Stay
There are 8 water-soluble B vitamins as well as vitamin C.

	Adult Men	Adult Women	Breastfeeding Women
Vitamin B1 (thiamine)	1.2 mg	1.1 mg	1.7 mg
Vitamin B2 (riboflavin)	1.3 mg	1.1 mg	2.0 mg
Vitamin B3 (niacin)	**16.0 mg**	**14.0 mg**	**20.0 mg**
Vitamin B5 (pantothenic acid)	5.0 mg	5.0 mg	10.0 mg
Vitamin B6 (pyridoxine)	1.3 mg	1.3 mg	2.0 mg
Vitamin B7 (biotin)	30 mcg	30 mcg	300 mcg
Vitamin B9 (folic acid, folate)	400 mcg	400 mcg	800 mcg
Vitamin B12 (cobalamin)	2.4 mcg	2.4 mcg	8.0 mcg
Vitamin C	90 mg	75 mg	120 mg

Table 7. RDA for the 8 Water-Soluble Vitamins

Except for Niacin (Vitamin B3), there are no known side effects or toxicity at high doses. The common side effect of too much Vitamin B3 is diarrhea, nausea, and abdominal cramps.

Taking too much vitamin C will not kill you. Around 2,000mg of vitamin C is considered the limit before you start getting headaches. However, anything over 1,000mg can cause diarrhea.

These vitamins enhance the enzymes that help us digest and absorb nutrients in our bodies. Your body doesn't store water-soluble vitamins except for vitamin B12. So, eating a balanced diet with lots of microgreens every day should get you what you need.

When to Be Cautious

However, there is a reason why you only see rhubarb stalks at your grocery. Rhubarb leaves contain oxalic acid, which is used in bleach and antirust products! Overeat and you might start to vomit and feel weak.

But don't worry. The research I found says if you're about 145 pounds (65.7 kg), it will take about 25 grams (0.06 lbs.) of pure oxalic acid to kill you. You'd need to eat about 11 pounds (5 kg) of rhubarb leaves, and 7 pounds (3.2 kg) of spinach at one sitting to get that 24 grams of oxalic acid.

But the central debate about oxalic acid in food is whether it can give you kidney stones.

But just about every leafy green vegetable contains oxalic acid. Spinach has the highest levels of oxalic acid–750 milligrams per 100-gram serving. So, do you need to worry? Nope, not at all.

While they are packed with nutrients essential to our health, spinach, beet, and Swiss chard microgreens are also high in oxalic acid. It is the source of their slightly bitter taste. In moderation, they are fine, though.

Microgreens and Bad Body Odor

You have two types of sweat glands: *the eccrine and apocrine glands.*

The eccrine gland makes odorless sweat (mainly sodium chloride) to lower body temperature.

The apocrine glands sit in your armpits, groin, and scalp and produce fatty sweat that mixes with bacteria, which causes an unpleasant odor.

Also, the food you eat, as it is broken down by your body, can react with the skin bacteria and further change your body odor.

I couldn't find a lot of research pointing to microgreens and body odor. Still, there's enough information out there to give you an idea of what kinds of foods could change your body odor.

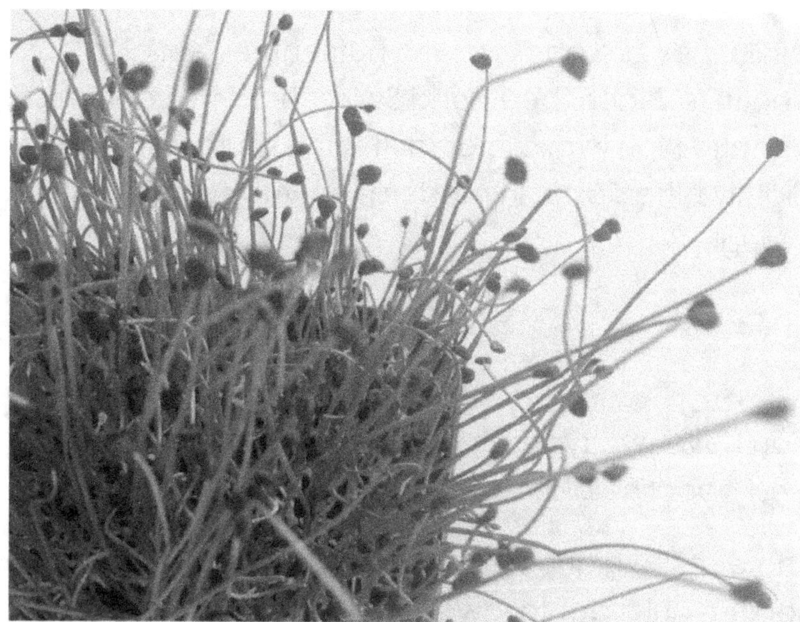

Figure 2. Onion Microgreens

Garlic Chives Microgreens

You're certainly not going to eat garlic anything before a date or interview. But did you know this? Rub crushed garlic on your feet, then wait 30 minutes. You will taste the garlic in your mouth. Wondering why?

Your feet are filled with tiny blood vessels that absorb allicin, the main compound in garlic. Allicin turns into sulfur compounds that find their way into your lungs and give you that stinking smell.

Onions Microgreens

Onions also break down into sulfur compounds.

But onion microgreens never make you cry - even if you chop them!

Cruciferous Microgreens

Cabbage, bok choy or Chinese cabbage, and broccoli, for example, also contain ample amounts of sulfur in the form of sulforaphane.

But you'd have to eat a ton (well maybe several pounds) to change body odor (through your breath, sweat, or farting).

Curry, cumin and other microgreen spices

From what I've read, it seems that people who eat lots of curries have body odors that smell like these spice aromas.

So, if you plan on eating potentially smelly microgreens, you may want to take note that you could smell.

Your Antidote

I've seen where drinking milk before or after removes the smell. But chlorophyll, the thing that makes plants bright green, is a <u>natural body deodorant</u>.

Funny, isn't it.

Eat chlorophyll-rich microgreens such as spinach and watercress to counter the smell of broccoli and garlic chives odors.

Which Ones Should I Eat?

Here are five varieties of microgreens that you can eat daily at every meal and not worry about overeating or eating too little.

Broccoli microgreens contain more than 550% of the RDA of antioxidant nutrients you need. It has the most complete nutrient profile of any vegetable.

It is packed with Vitamin A, B, C and K, and a sizeable amount of iron, magnesium, and phosphorus.

Kale microgreens are one of the latest food trends.

It has a lower antioxidant capacity than broccoli. Still, it has more vitamin B, just as much vitamin C, but less vitamin A than broccoli.

Pea shoot microgreens are an antioxidant like broccoli. Though not as high in nutritional quality as kale or microgreens, eaten together with those two, it delivers a lot of vitamin B's: *B3(niacin), B1 (thiamin), B2 (riboflavin), B-6 (pyridoxine) and B9 (folate)*.

They also have double the concentration of iron, phosphorus, and magnesium compared to broccoli.

Radish microgreens are the forgotten part of the radish.

Most people eat the root or bulb. It is in the same family as broccoli and kale, Brassicaceae (or mustard), and contains a different set of vitamins and minerals, including magnesium, zinc, and phosphorus.

And last but not least, **amaranth microgreens**, which includes quinoa, is very well balanced in nutrients that include little of Vitamin A, B, and C, and a significant source of minerals such as calcium, iron, and magnesium.

Of all the other microgreens, amaranth has the highest antioxidant capacity.

Eat To Meet Your RDA
Rotating microgreens and other foods regularly help to limit the over-consumption of anti-nutrients and provides health-promoting variety in your diet. Also, by adding microgreens to your meals, you will help to close any gaps in your vitamin or mineral intake.

Learn a lot more about microgreens, how good they are for you, and what you can do with them. Check out my guide, "The Beginner's Nutritional Guide to Incredible Microgreens."

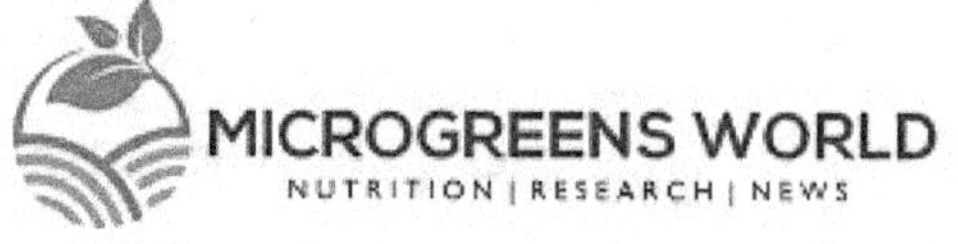

Visit Microgreens World: http://microgreensworld.com/

BAHAMIAN CONCH SOUP WITH CILANTRO MICROGREENS

Most Caribbean islands have a national recipe, and conch is the specialty cuisine of the Grand Bahamas. Conch comes in three different varieties: *queen, king, and horse.*

Microgreen	Taste	Aroma	Flavor	Intensity
Cilantro	Lemony		Citrus	Strong

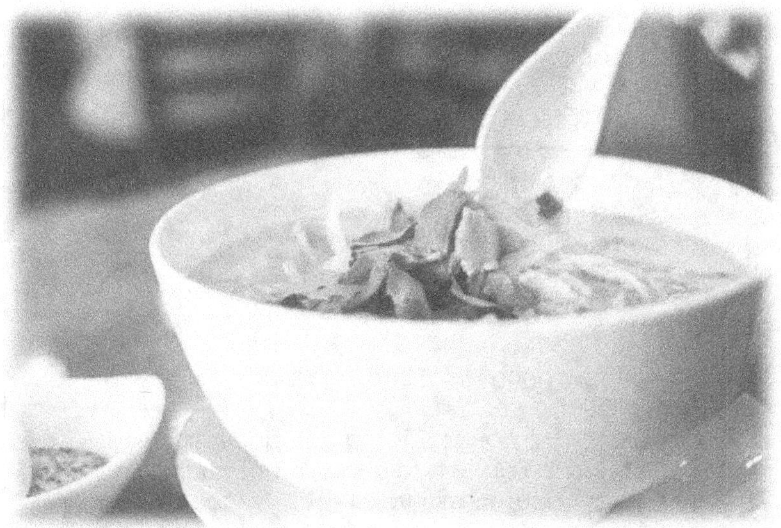

With a hint of sweetness like a scallop, the locals consider conch soup to be a potent aphrodisiac.

You can order yours from Giovanni's Fish Market.

Bahamian Conch and Cilantro Microgreens Soup

Prep Time	50 mins

Course: Soup

Cuisine: Bahamian

Keyword: conch, cilantro microgreens

Servings: 4 people   Calories: 150 kcal

Equipment

- 4-quart Soup Pot

Ingredients

- 2 oz cilantro microgreens
- 1 cup conch meat
- 1 qt. of water
- 1/2 lb. diced tomatoes
- 1/2 lb. sliced onions
- 2 tablespoons oil
- * herbs, garlic, salt to taste
- 1 tsp sherry (optional)

Instructions

1. Chop the conch meat into cubes and boil in water for about 30 minutes.
2. Heat oil and fry onions, tomatoes, and seasonings.
3. Add these ingredients to conch meat and liquid.
4. Cook for about 15 minutes.
5. Add microgreens and cook for 5 more minutes
6. Add a teaspoon sherry an aromatic taste.

Note: Only the meat of the *young queen conch* must be used.

Nutrition Facts

Serving size: 2 cups

Servings: 4

Amount per serving

Calories 150

% Daily Value*

Total Fat 8g	10%
Saturated Fat 1.2g	6%
Cholesterol 165mg	55%
Sodium 259mg	11%
Total Carbohydrate 8.5g	3%
Dietary Fiber 2.2g	8%
Total Sugars 4.2g	
Protein 12.4g	
Vitamin D 0mcg	0%
Calcium 44mg	3%
Iron 1mg	6%
Potassium 294mg	6%

*The % Daily Value (DV) tells you how much a nutrient in a food serving contributes to a daily diet. 2,000 calorie a day is used for general nutrition advice.

Recipe analyzed by very**well**

TRINI PUMPKIN AND CHAYOTE SOUP WITH BOK CHOY MICROGREENS

<u>Chayote</u> is a pear-shaped, light green vegetable belonging to the gourd family. It is prevalent in Latin America and the Caribbean, including Trinidad.

It is a rich source of dietary fiber, magnesium, phosphorus, potassium, vitamin C, and choline.

Microgreen	Taste	Aroma	Flavor	Intensity
Bok Choy	Sweet	Juicy	Earthy	Mild

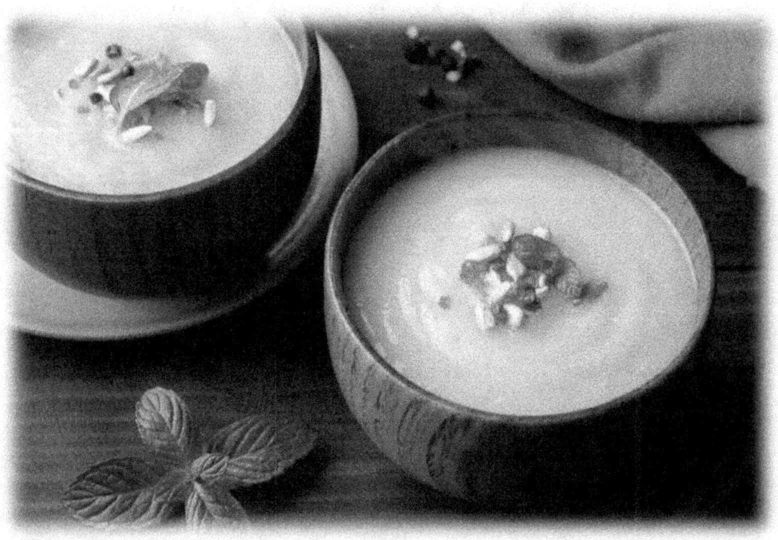

<u>Bok choy</u> microgreens add a cabbage-like flavor and crisp texture to the soup.

Trini Pumpkin and Chayote Soup with Bok Choy Microgreens

Prep Time	30 mins

Course: **Soup**   Cuisine: **Caribbean**   Keyword: **bok choy microgreens**

Servings: **4 people**   Calories: **135 kcal**

Equipment

- 4-Quart Soup pot.

Ingredients

- 4 oz bok choy microgreens
- 1 lb (450 g) pumpkin
- 1 Chayote
- 11/2 pt (800 ml) water
- 2 medium-sized tomatoes
- 1 spring onion
- 1 sprig thyme
- 1 small blade mace
- ½ tsp freshly ground black pepper
- 1/4 pints (150 ml) coconut milk

Instructions

1. Peel and wash the pumpkin.
2. Remove the seeds and chop into 2 cm dice.
3. Peel the chayote, cut into quarters lengthways, and remove the heart. Dice.
4. Place the pumpkin and the chayote in a saucepan with the water and simmer on medium heat for 15 minutes or until cooked.
5. Meanwhile, peel and chop the tomatoes and microgreens.
6. Slice the spring onion into fine rounds. Add these to the saucepan together with the thyme, mace, ground black pepper, and coconut milk.
7. Simmer for a further 15 minutes then remove the thyme before serving.

Nutrition Facts

Serving size: 2 cups

Servings: 4

Amount per serving

Calories 135

% Daily Value*

Total Fat 7.8g	10%
Saturated Fat 6.6g	33%
Cholesterol 0mg	0%
Sodium 49mg	2%
Total Carbohydrate 16.8g	6%
Dietary Fiber 6.1g	22%
Total Sugars 7.5g	
Protein 3.4g	
Vitamin D 0mcg	0%
Calcium 101mg	8%
Iron 3mg	17%
Potassium 599mg	13%

*The % Daily Value (DV) tells you how much a nutrient in a food serving contributes to a daily diet. 2,000 calorie a day is used for general nutrition advice.

Recipe analyzed by very**well**

JAMAICAN RED AND FAVA BEAN MICROGREEN SOUP

Red peas soup is a Saturday lunch meal found in most island venues like Jamaica. Rich in phytonutrients, this seemingly humble bean is a nutritional powerhouse.

Microgreen	Taste	Aroma	Flavor	Intensity
Fava Bean	Sweet	Juicy	Nutty	Crunchy

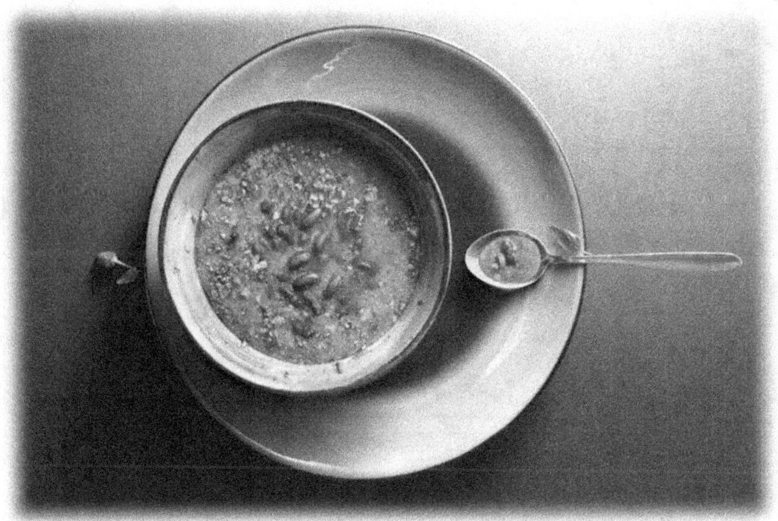

The combination of red beans, fava beans, and different colored vegetables makes this a visually attractive as well as a nourishing soup.

Jamaican Kidney and Fava Bean Microgreen Soup

Prep Time	35 mins

Course: Soup

Cuisine: Caribbean

Keyword: fava beans microgreens

Servings: 4 people   **Calories:** 490 kcal

Equipment

- 4-5-quart Soup pot; Skillet.

Ingredients

- 2 oz fava bean microgreens
- 1 lb (450 g) red (kidney) beans (pre-cooked)
- 2 pt (1100 ml) water
- 1 large onion
- 1 medium-sized carrot
- 1 stick celery
- 1 green pepper
- 2 tbs vegetable oil
- 2 cloves garlic
- 1 Scotch Bonnet pepper
- 1 sprig thyme
- freshly ground black pepper

Instructions

1. Open the can of red beans and set aside.
2. Peel and finely chop the onion.
3. Peel and slice the carrot.
4. Chop the celery and green pepper.
5. In a separate pan, heat the vegetable oil.
6. Add the chopped vegetables and the crushed cloves of garlic.
7. Cook gently until soft for about 10 min.
8. Crush some of the cooked red beans with their liquid to make a coarse purée.
9. Pour the two pints of water into the soup pot.
10. Add the red bean purée, and the remaining beans to the pot. Stir.
11. Add the whole Scotch Bonnet pepper, thyme and black pepper.
12. Simmer for 15 minutes.
13. Add the fava bean microgreens and cook for 5 minutes more.
14. Remove thyme and whole pepper before serving.
15. Serve hot.

Nutrition Facts

Serving size: 2 cups

Servings: 4

Amount per serving

Calories 490

% Daily Value*

Total Fat 8.2g	**11%**
Saturated Fat 1.5g	**8%**
Cholesterol 0mg	**0%**
Sodium 44mg	**2%**
Total Carbohydrate 79.9g	**29%**
Dietary Fiber 20g	**71%**
Total Sugars 6.4g	
Protein 27.6g	
Vitamin D 0mcg	0%
Calcium 135mg	10%
Iron 8mg	47%
Potassium 1798mg	38%

*The % Daily Value (DV) tells you how much a nutrient in a food serving contributes to a daily diet. 2,000 calorie a day is used for general nutrition advice.

Recipe analyzed by very**well**

BELIZE CALLALOO AND MUSTARD MICROGREENS SOUP

Callaloo (amaranth) is a popular and indigenous Caribbean vegetable and is another nutrient-packed food.

When paired with mustard microgreens, you get an array of vitamins, including E, thiamin, B6, riboflavin, and niacin, and minerals, including manganese and selenium.

Microgreen	Taste	Aroma	Flavor	Intensity
Mustard	Sweet		Spicy	High

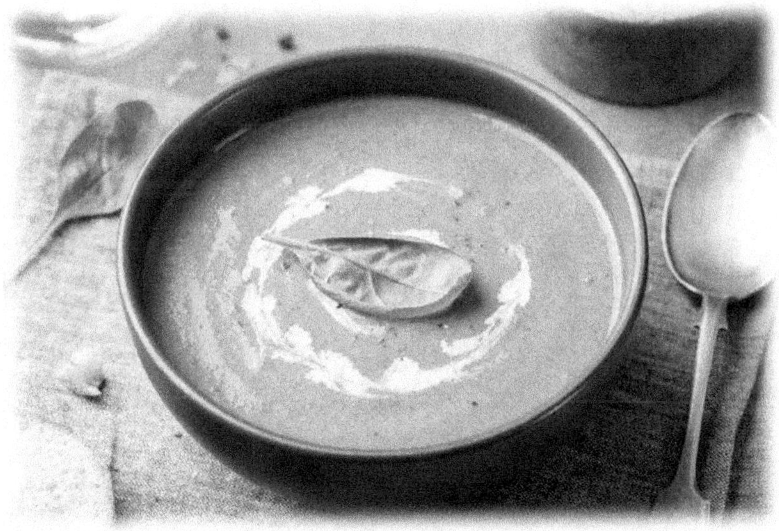

With a salad and whole wheat bread, this soup becomes a meal.

Belize Callaloo and Mustard Microgreens Soup

Prep Time	40 mins

Course: Soup

Cuisine: Caribbean

Keyword: callaloo, mustard microgreens

Servings: 4 people   Calories: 235 kcal

Equipment

- 14 oz Soup Pan

Ingredients

- 4 oz mustard microgreens
- 1 lb (450 g) callaloo leaves
- 1 aubergine (eggplant)
- 2 green bananas
- 1 large onion
- 2 cloves garlic
- 11/2 pts (850 ml) water
- 4 pimento berries
- 3 whole cloves
- 1 sprig thyme
- 1 hot pepper
- freshly ground black pepper
- 1/2 lb (225 g) young okra
- 1/4 pt (150 ml) coconut milk

Instructions

1. Thoroughly wash the callaloo leaves and remove most of the stem. Drain and coarsely chop.
2. Peel the eggplant and chop into 2 cm dice.
3. Keeping the skin on, cut the green bananas into thick slices.
4. Place these vegetables together with chopped onion and garlic in a large soup pan.
5. Add the water, pimento, cloves, thyme, hot pepper, and freshly ground black pepper.
6. Bring the soup to a boil and simmer, covered until the vegetables are tender.
7. Take out the slices of green banana, remove the skin, and return to the pan.
8. Remove the hot pepper, which should still be whole and the thyme.
9. Rub the soup through a sieve or liquidize briefly.
10. Slice the okra into rounds.
11. Return the soup to the pan.
12. Add the okra, coconut milk, and microgreens.
13. Cook for a further 10 minutes.
14. Adjust the seasoning and serve.

Note: If it is more readily available, use spinach as a substitute for callaloo.

Nutrition Facts

Serving size: 2 cups
Servings: 4

Amount per serving
Calories 235

% Daily Value*

Total Fat 8.1g	10%
Saturated Fat 6.5g	33%
Cholesterol 0mg	0%
Sodium 687mg	30%
Total Carbohydrate 39.5g	14%
Dietary Fiber 12.9g	46%
Total Sugars 20.5g	
Protein 6.8g	
Vitamin D 0mcg	0%
Calcium 111mg	9%
Iron 4mg	21%
Potassium 804mg	17%

*The % Daily Value (DV) tells you how much a nutrient in a food serving contributes to a daily diet. 2,000 calorie a day is used for general nutrition advice.

Recipe analyzed by very**well**

SOUTHWESTERN SWEETCORN AND PARSLEY MICROGREENS SOUP

Parsley microgreens are excellent to flavor most any dish. Parsley is the world's most popular herb, high in magnesium, phosphorus, potassium, sodium, and all the essential vitamins, especially K content.

Microgreen	Taste	Aroma	Flavor	Intensity
Parsley	Sweet		Fruity	Mild

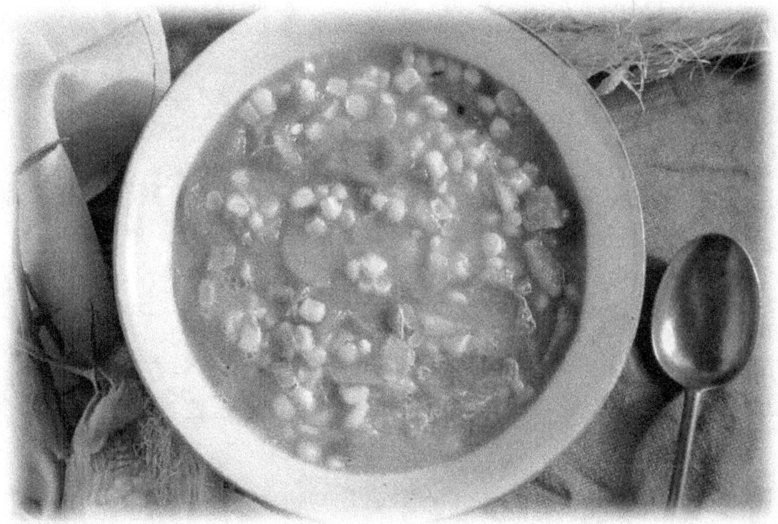

A creamy vegetable soup thickened with potato and pumpkin. Serve with a simple salad or whole wheat bread.

Southwestern Sweetcorn and Parsley Microgreens Soup

Prep Time	55 mins

Course: Soup

Cuisine: Southwestern US

Keyword: parsley microgreens

Servings: 4 people   Calories: 481 kcal

Equipment

- 4-Quart Soup pot

Ingredients

- 4 oz parsley microgreens
- 8 oz (225 g) sweetcorn
- 11/2 pt (850 ml) water
- 1/3 pt (200 ml) coconut milk
- 2 medium-sized potatoes
- 1 lb (450g) pumpkin
- 1 stick celery
- 2 spring onions
- 1 medium-sized tomato
- 1 sprig thyme
- freshly ground black pepper to taste
- juice of 1/2 lime

Instructions

1. Place the corn in a heavy-based soup pot
2. Cover with water, bring to the boil and simmer.
3. Peel the potatoes and pumpkin remove the pumpkin seeds and dice both vegetables.
4. Chop the celery and spring onions, peel, and chop the tomato.
5. Add the coconut milk to the pot together with the prepared vegetables.
6. Season with thyme and freshly ground black pepper and add the lime juice.
7. Continue to cook on a low heat for 15-20 minutes until the vegetables are soft.
8. Add the microgreens and cook for 5-10 more minutes
9. Remove the thyme before serving.

Nutrition Facts

Serving size: 2 cups
Servings: 4

Amount per serving
Calories 481

% Daily Value*

Total Fat 13.7g	**18%**
Saturated Fat 9.3g	**46%**
Cholesterol 0mg	**0%**
Sodium 99mg	**4%**
Total Carbohydrate 88.8g	**32%**
Dietary Fiber 16.2g	**58%**
Total Sugars 17.5g	
Protein 14.7g	
Vitamin D 0mcg	0%
Calcium 93mg	7%
Iron 12mg	66%
Potassium 1775mg	38%

*The % Daily Value (DV) tells you how much a nutrient in a food serving contributes to a daily diet. 2,000 calorie a day is used for general nutrition advice.

Recipe analyzed by very**well**

MEXICAN BEET MICROGREENS SOUP

Types of beet such as Bulls Blood or Rainbow are grown for their intense red color on even very young seedlings.

Microgreen	Taste	Aroma	Flavor	Intensity
Beet	Sweet		Earthy	Mild

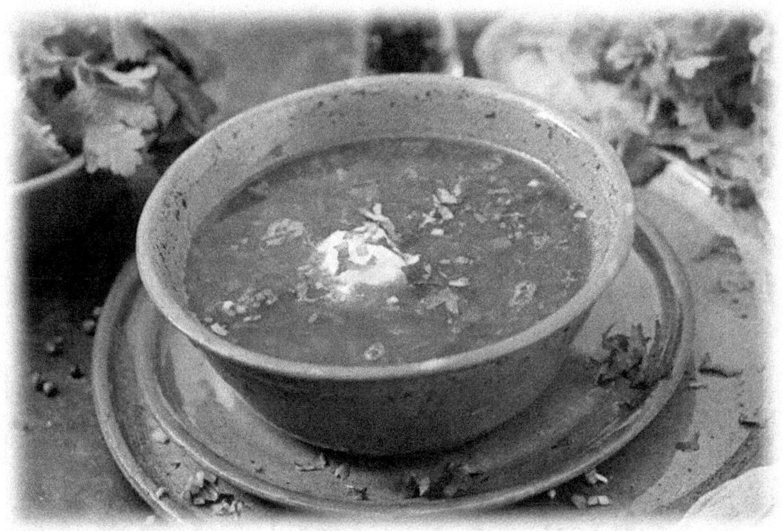

Add an extra sprinkle of salt to highlight their sweetness, and you have rich and nutritious meal.

Mexican Beet Microgreens Soup

Prep Time	1 hour 45 mins

Course: Soup   Cuisine: Latin American   Keyword: beet microgreens

Servings: 4 people   Calories: 194 kcal

Equipment

- 4-Quart Soup pot.

Ingredients

- 2 oz beet microgreens rinsed and dried
- 8 large cooked and peeled beets
- 1lb. soup meat cut into cubes
- 3 diced tomatoes
- 2 qt water
- 1 cup shredded cabbage
- salt, pepper, and sour cream

Instructions

1. Combine meat, tomatoes, and water in a soup pot.
2. Bring to a boil.
3. Skim and cook for about an hour
4. Add the cabbage, salt, and pepper. Cook for 30 minutes.
5. Grate the beetroots and add to the soup with salt and pepper. Cook for 15 min.
6. Add microgreens and stir.
7. Serve very hot, with a spoonful of sour cream and a few pieces of the meat in each soup bowl.

Nutrition Facts

Serving size: 2 cups

Servings: 4

Amount per serving

Calories 194

% Daily Value*

Total Fat 4.2g	5%
Saturated Fat 1.4g	7%
Cholesterol 51mg	17%
Sodium 804mg	35%
Total Carbohydrate 18.1g	7%
Dietary Fiber 9.2g	33%
Total Sugars 3.3g	
Protein 25.1g	
Vitamin D 0mcg	0%
Calcium 358mg	28%
Iron 16mg	91%
Potassium 2929mg	62%

*The % Daily Value (DV) tells you how much a nutrient in a food serving contributes to a daily diet. 2,000 calorie a day is used for general nutrition advice.

Recipe analyzed by **very**well

BELIZE CHAYOTE AND CARROT MICROGREENS SOUP

Chayote is a rich source of dietary fiber, magnesium, phosphorus, potassium, vitamin C, and choline. Carrot microgreens are a superbly rich source of antioxidants, carotenes, and vitamin A.

Microgreen	Taste	Aroma	Flavor	Intensity
Carrot	Sweet		Crunchy	Mild

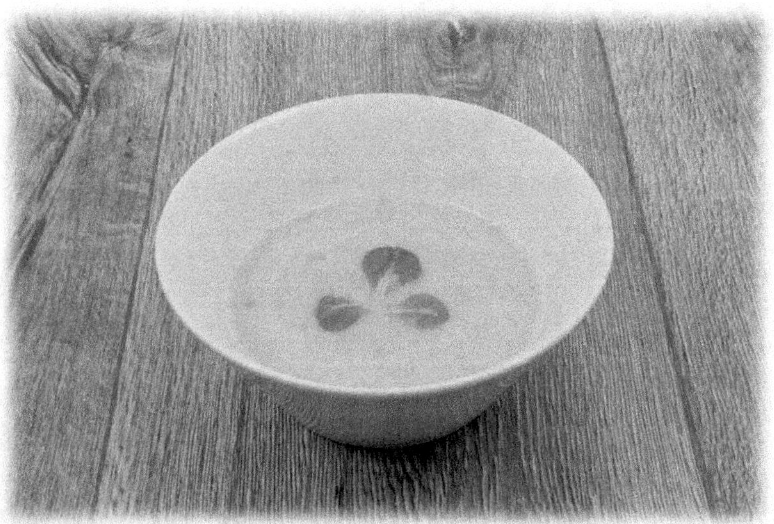

Together they provide a creamy, rich soup to fill any afternoon appetite.

Belize Chayote and Carrot Microgreens Soup

Prep Time	30 mins

Course:
Soup

Cuisine:
Caribbean

Keyword: carrot
microgreens

Servings: 4 people   Calories: 80 kcal

Equipment

- 3 Quart Soup Pan.

Ingredients

- 4 oz carrot microgreens rinsed and dried
- 4 chayote peeled and diced
- 1 cup milk
- * butter, herbs, salt, nutmeg to taste

Instructions

1. Boil chayote until tender.
2. Pour into blender with herbs and milk and blend until smooth.
3. Chop and add microgreens.
4. Reheat to serve with a dab of butter and pinch of nutmeg.

Nutrition Facts

Serving size: 2 cups
Servings: 4

Amount per serving

Calories 80

% Daily Value*

Total Fat 1.7g	2%
Saturated Fat 0.9g	5%
Cholesterol 5mg	2%
Sodium 56mg	2%
Total Carbohydrate 14.5g	5%
Dietary Fiber 4.3g	**15%**
Total Sugars 7.5g	
Protein 3.8g	
Vitamin D 0mcg	2%
Calcium 116mg	9%
Iron 1mg	5%
Potassium 356mg	8%

**The % Daily Value (DV) tells you how much a nutrient in a food serving contributes to a daily diet. 2,000 calorie a day is used for general nutrition advice.*

Recipe analyzed by **very**well

FLORIDA FISH TEA AND KALE MICROGREENS

Kale is a "superfood" capable of lowering bad cholesterol. It contains carotenoid antioxidants in high concentrations, which reduces the risk of eye problems (macular degeneration and cataracts).

Microgreen	Taste	Aroma	Flavor	Intensity
Kale	Slight Bitter		Crunchy	Mild

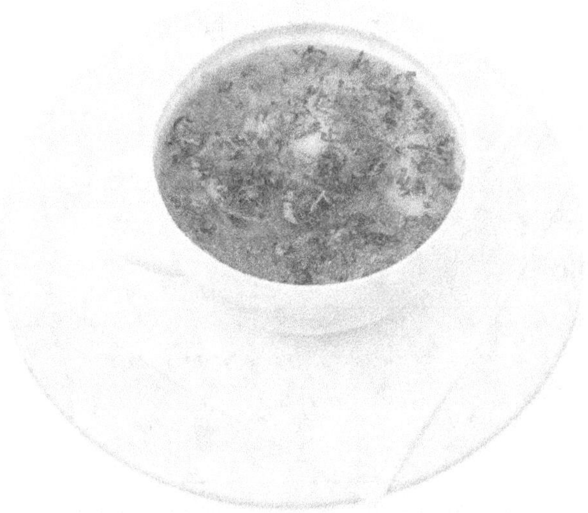

A traditional Friday evening soup on the docks. Excellent with red snapper and seasoned to perfection with selected herbs and spices.

Florida Fish Tea and Kale Microgreens

Prep Time	50 mins

Course: Soup

Cuisine: International

Keyword: kale microgreens

Servings: 4 people   Calories: 476 kcal

Equipment

- 4-Quart Soup pot. Large serving bowls.

Ingredients

- 2 oz kale microgreens rinsed and dried
- 3 lbs. of fish (snapper) cut into pieces
- 6 cups of water
- 2 chopped onions
- 2 chopped tomatoes
- 1 hot pepper
- 1 tsp. thyme
- * squeeze of lime juice

Instructions

1. Place all ingredients in a pot with water.
2. Bring to a boil and simmer gently for about 45 minutes.
3. Strain off liquid into serving bowl.
4. Serve over chopped kale microgreens.

Nutrition Facts

Serving size: 2 cups

Servings: 4

Amount per serving

Calories 476

	% Daily Value*
Total Fat 6.2g	8%
Saturated Fat 0g	0%
Cholesterol 160mg	53%
Sodium 218mg	9%
Total Carbohydrate 8.2g	3%
Dietary Fiber 2.1g	7%
Total Sugars 4g	
Protein 89.4g	
Vitamin D 0mcg	0%
Calcium 200mg	15%
Iron 2mg	12%
Potassium 253mg	5%

*The % Daily Value (DV) tells you how much a nutrient in a food serving contributes to a daily diet. 2,000 calorie a day is used for general nutrition advice.

Recipe analyzed by **very well**

SOUTHERN OLD-FASHIONED LENTIL MICROGREENS SOUP

Lentils have been in the human diet since prehistoric times. India and Canada are the largest producers.

Lentils microgreens are very rich in proteins, dietary fiber, minerals (copper, iron, and folate), and vitamins B and C.

Microgreen	Taste	Aroma	Flavor	Intensity
Lentils	Slightly Bitter			Mild

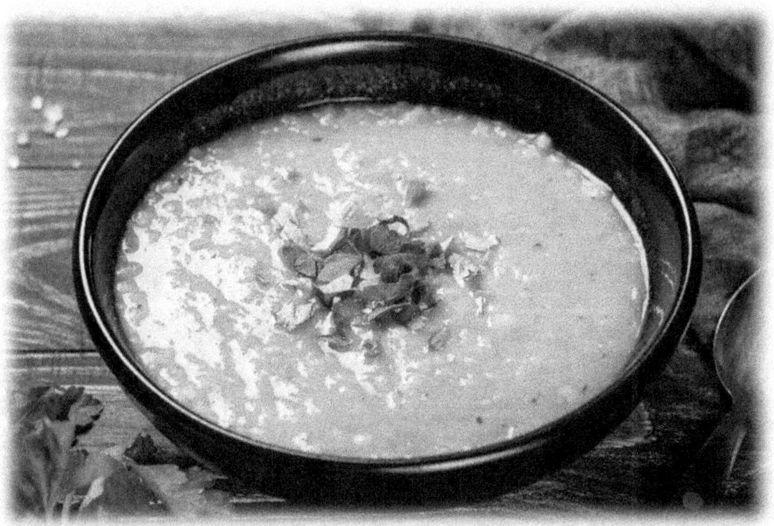

The main course meal is served with warm bread.

Southern Old-Fashioned Lentil Microgreens Soup

Prep Time	1 hr. 5 min.

Course: Soup

Cuisine: Southern USA

Keyword: lentil microgreens

Servings: 3 people

Calories: 145 kcal

Equipment

- 4 Quart Soup Kettle.

Ingredients

- 2 oz lentil microgreens rinsed and dried
- 71/2 cups water
- 1 clove garlic, minced
- 1 large white onion, chopped
- 2 large carrots, coarsely chopped
- 2 stalks celery, coarsely chopped
- 11/2 cups lentils
- 1 vegetable bouillon or 1 tablespoon red miso
- 1/2 teaspoon dried thyme
- 1 teaspoon dried oregano
- 1-2 tbsp fresh parsley, chopped
- 1 teaspoon sweet Hungarian paprika
- 1/2 teaspoon Spike (optional)
- 1/2 teaspoon sea salt (optional)
- 1 cup fresh or frozen corn (optional)

Instructions

1. In soup kettle, bring water to a boil.
2. Add garlic, onion, carrots, celery, lentils, and bouillon or miso.
3. Return to boil.
4. Add seasonings. Mix well.
5. Simmer covered over low heat for 60 minutes.
6. If you want a creamier consistency, you can puree 1/2 the soup in blender or food processor.
7. Stir in lentil microgreens.
8. Return to heat and add corn, if desired.
9. Simmer for 5 minutes.

Nutrition Facts

Serving size: cups

Servings: 3

Amount per serving

Calories 145

% Daily Value*

Total Fat 0.8g	1%
Saturated Fat 0.1g	1%
Cholesterol 0mg	0%
Sodium 66mg	3%
Total Carbohydrate 27.3g	10%
Dietary Fiber 5.3g	19%
Total Sugars 5.1g	
Protein 7.5g	
Vitamin D 0mcg	0%
Calcium 79mg	6%
Iron 3mg	16%
Potassium 480mg	10%

*The % Daily Value (DV) tells you how much a nutrient in a food serving contributes to a daily diet. 2,000 calorie a day is used for general nutrition advice.

Recipe analyzed by very**well**

SOUTHWESTERN GOLDEN POTATO AND PARSLEY MICROGREENS SOUP

Potatoes are low in calories, about 110 when boiled, and a good source of vitamins C and B6, manganese, phosphorus, niacin, and pantothenic acid.

Microgreen	Taste	Aroma	Flavor	Intensity
Parsley	Sweet		Fruity	Mild

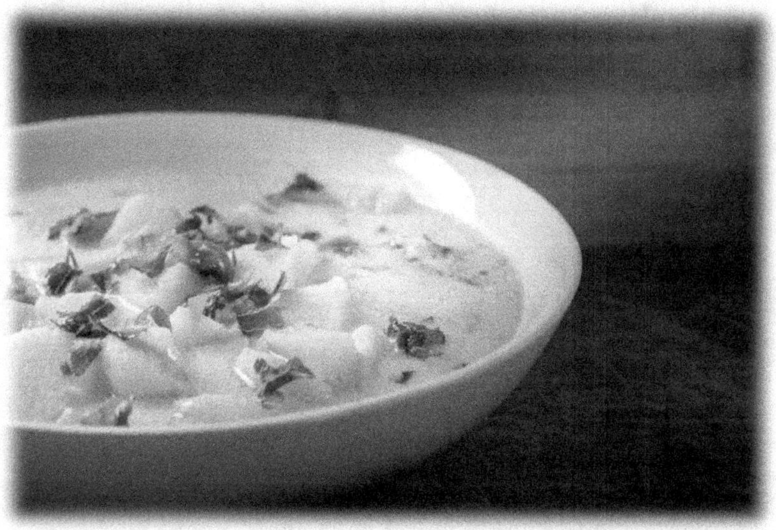

This international staple, when paired with parsley microgreens, is a "superfood" meal on its own. Just add fresh bread and a glass of Chablis.

Southwestern Golden Potato and Parsley Microgreens Soup

Prep Time	30 mins

Course: Soup

Cuisine: Southwestern US

Keyword: parsley microgreens

Servings: 4 people

Calories: 304 kcal

Equipment

- 4-5 Quart Soup pot. Blender.

Ingredients

- 2 oz parsley microgreens rinsed and dried
- 2 tablespoons butter
- 1 tsp safflower oil
- 1 clove garlic, minced
- 1 large onion, coarsely chopped
- 2 cups celery, chopped
- 5 medium russet potatoes or 8 White Rose potatoes, peeled and cut into 1-inch cubes
- 6-8 crookneck squash, cut into 1-inch slices
- 1 tablespoon white miso or 1 vegetable bouillon
- 1 teaspoon dried thyme
- 1/4 teaspoon dried tarragon
- 1/2 teaspoon dried sage
- Sea salt, seasoned salt, or salt-free seasoning to taste
- Dash of cayenne to taste
- 6-7 cups water

Instructions

1. In heavy soup kettle, melt butter and heat oil.
2. Add garlic, onion, celery, and sauté until the ingredients begin to wilt.
3. Add potatoes, squash, miso or bouillon, and seasoning.
4. Add water to cover vegetables.
5. Bring to a boil, simmer covered for 20 minutes, or until vegetables are soft.
6. Cool slightly and puree in increments in the blender to a smooth golden cream.
7. Add microgreens to the pot.
8. Reheat gently, stirring, so the soup doesn't stick.
9. Serve warm with crackers or whole wheat bread.

Nutrition Facts

Serving size: 2 cups

Servings: 4

Amount per serving

Calories 304

% Daily Value*

Total Fat 7.7g	10%
Saturated Fat 3.9g	19%
Cholesterol 15mg	5%
Sodium 370mg	16%
Total Carbohydrate 53.4g	19%
Dietary Fiber 10.1g	36%
Total Sugars 8.7g	
Protein 7.5g	
Vitamin D 4mcg	20%
Calcium 81mg	6%
Iron 3mg	16%
Potassium 1321mg	28%

*The % Daily Value (DV) tells you how much a nutrient in a food serving contributes to a daily diet. 2,000 calorie a day is used for general nutrition advice.

Recipe analyzed by very**well**

CARIBBEAN CAULIFLOWER AND SWEET PEA MICROGREEN SOUP

One serving of cauliflower has 100% of your RDA of vitamin C ,and 25% of vitamin K.

In addition to 50% of your Vitamin C RDA, sweet pea microgreens have concentrated nutrition and blood cleansing properties.

Microgreen	Taste	Aroma	Flavor	Intensity
Sweet Pea	Sweet		Crunchy	Mild

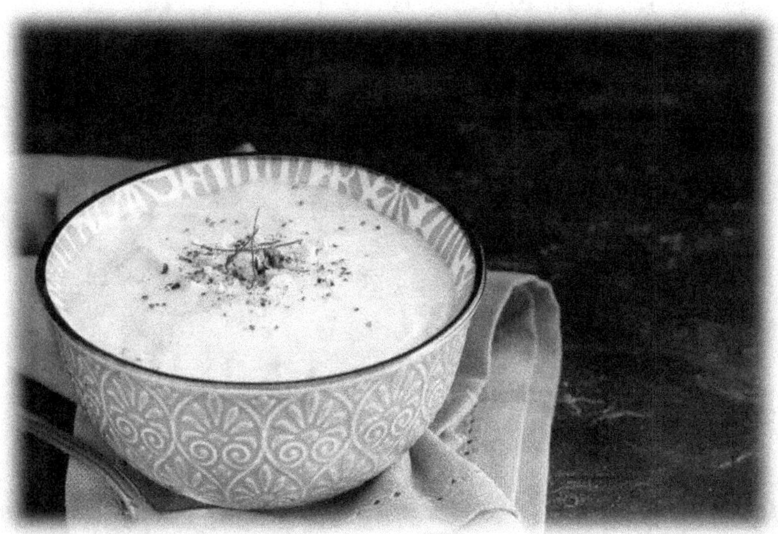

A power-packed Vitamin C meal for fighting infections.

Caribbean Cauliflower and Sugar Pea Microgreens Soup

Prep Time	35 mins

Course:
Soup

Cuisine:
American

Keywords:
sweet pea microgreens

Servings: 3 people   Calories: 135 kcal

Equipment

- 3-Quart Soup kettle. Food processor

Ingredients

- 3 oz sugar pea microgreens   rinsed and dried
- 5 cups of water
- 1 medium white onion, coarsely chopped
- 1 stalk celery, chopped
- 2 scallions, chopped
- 1 medium cauliflower, cored and cut into 1-inch florets
- 1 tablespoon white miso or I vegetable bouillon
- 2 cups fresh or frozen sugar peas
- 1 tablespoon fresh parsley, chopped
- 1teaspoon dried basil
- 1/4 teaspoon dried sage
- 2 teaspoons butter
- 1tsp sea salt (optional)
- 1/4 cup fresh cilantro, chopped (optional)
- 1/2 tsp seasoned salt or salt-free seasoning (optional)

Instructions

1. In heavy soup kettle, bring water to a boil.
2. Add onion celery, scallions, cauliflower, salt, and miso.
3. Return to boil. Simmer, covered, for 10 minutes.
4. Add Peas, dill parsley, basil, sage, and cilantro.
5. Return to boil, cover. Let simmer for an additional 10 minutes.
6. Remove cover, and cool slightly.
7. Puree in blender or food processor until creamy.
8. Return to heat. Add microgreens and butter and stir as you reheat.
9. Adjust seasonings, adding salt if desired.

NOTE: If you wish a chunky soup, you can reserve 2 cups of vegetables from the broth before pureeing and return them to the soup as you reheat.

Nutrition Facts

Serving size: cups
Servings: 3

Amount per serving

Calories   135

% Daily Value*

Total Fat 3.1g	**4%**
Saturated Fat 1.7g	**9%**
Cholesterol 7mg	**2%**
Sodium 308mg	**13%**
Total Carbohydrate 21.2g	**8%**
Dietary Fiber 7.5g	**27%**
Total Sugars 8.3g	
Protein 7.3g	
Vitamin D 2mcg	9%
Calcium 104mg	8%
Iron 2mg	10%
Potassium 648mg	14%

*The % Daily Value (DV) tells you how much a nutrient in a food serving contributes to a daily diet. 2,000 calorie a day is used for general nutrition advice.

Recipe analyzed by very**well**

EATING YOUR MICROGREENS EVERY DAY

Ready to eat your microgreens?

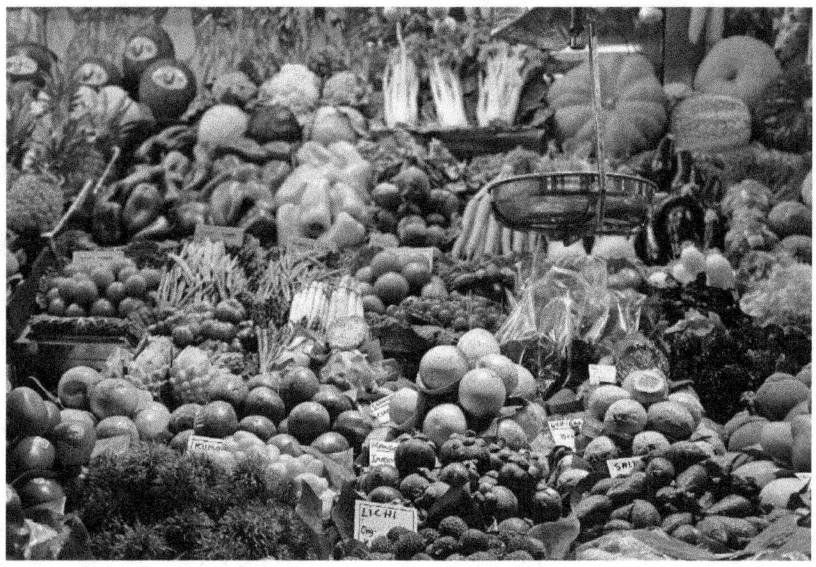

They are harvested right after germination and are packed with concentrated nutrients.

Until recently, commercially grown microgreens have only been available to chefs, who use them as flavor accents and garnishes for soups, salads, and sandwiches.

Today, they are available at farmer's markets and upscale grocery stores. They cost more than mature greens but have over 10 times the goodness.

Commercial Name	Family	Plant Color
Amaranth	Amaranthaceae	red
Celery	Apiaceae	green
Cilantro	Apiaceae	green
Arugula	Brassicaceae	green
Broccoli	Brassicaceae	green
Green Daikon Radish	Brassicaceae	purplish-green
Radish	Brassicaceae	green
Mizuna	Brassicaceae	green
Purple kohlrabi	Brassicaceae	purplish-green
Purple mustard	Brassicaceae	purplish-green
Opal radish	Brassicaceae	greenish-purple
Peppercress	Brassicaceae	green
Red cabbage	Brassicaceae	purplish-green
Red mustard	Brassicaceae	purplish-green
Wasabi	Brassicaceae	green
Beet	Chenopodiaceae	reddish-green
Magenta Spinach	Chenopodiaceae	red
Red beet	Chenopodiaceae	reddish-green
Red orach (arrach)	Chenopodiaceae	red
Pea tendrils	Fabaceae	green
Basil	Lamiaceae	green
Opal basil	Lamiaceae	greenish-purple
Popcorn shoots	Poaceae	yellow
Red sorrel	Polygonaceae	reddish-green
Sorrel	Polygonaceae	green

Table 8. Popular Commercially Sold Microgreens

And once you smell those intense flavors, absorb those bright colors, and bite into the tender textures of microgreens, you will be adding them as a garnish to your main meals, and enhancing your salads, soups, omelets, and sandwiches.

Learn a lot more about microgreens, how good they are for you, and what you can do with them. Check out my guide, "The Beginner's Nutritional Guide to Incredible Microgreens."

."
.

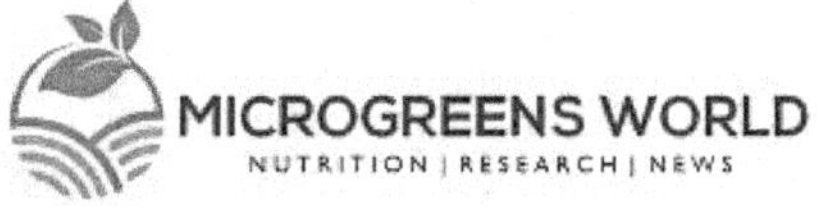

Visit Microgreens World: www.microgreensworld.com

WOULD YOU LEAVE A REVIEW?

As an author, I highly appreciate the feedback I get from my readers.

It helps others to make informed decisions before buying or reading my book.

If you enjoyed this book, please consider leaving a short review at the following link: **Leave A Review**

Want More Free Books?

Andrew Neves is giving away a free starter library

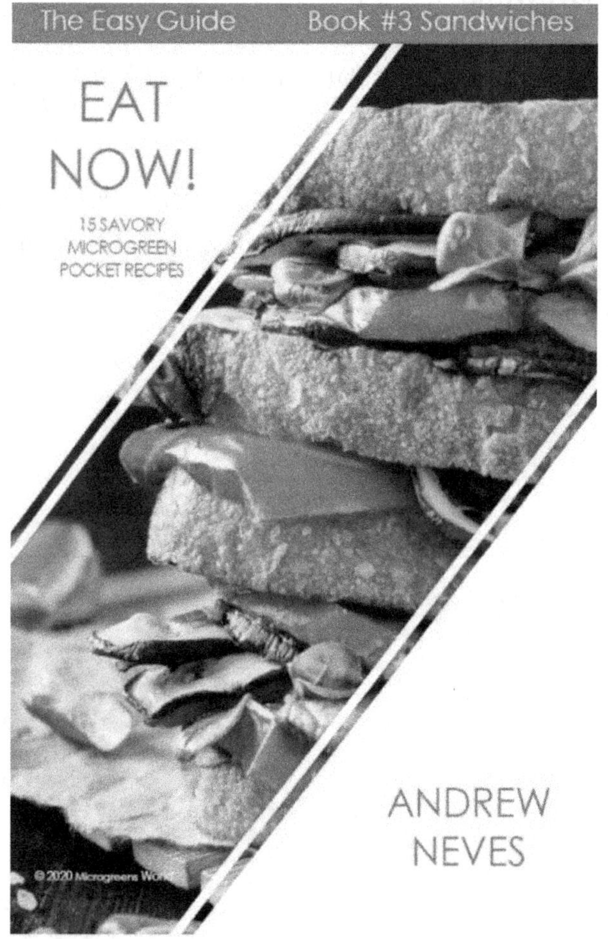

If you like **FREE**, then <u>CLICK HERE TO SIGN UP FOR FREE</u>

Get This Free Book!

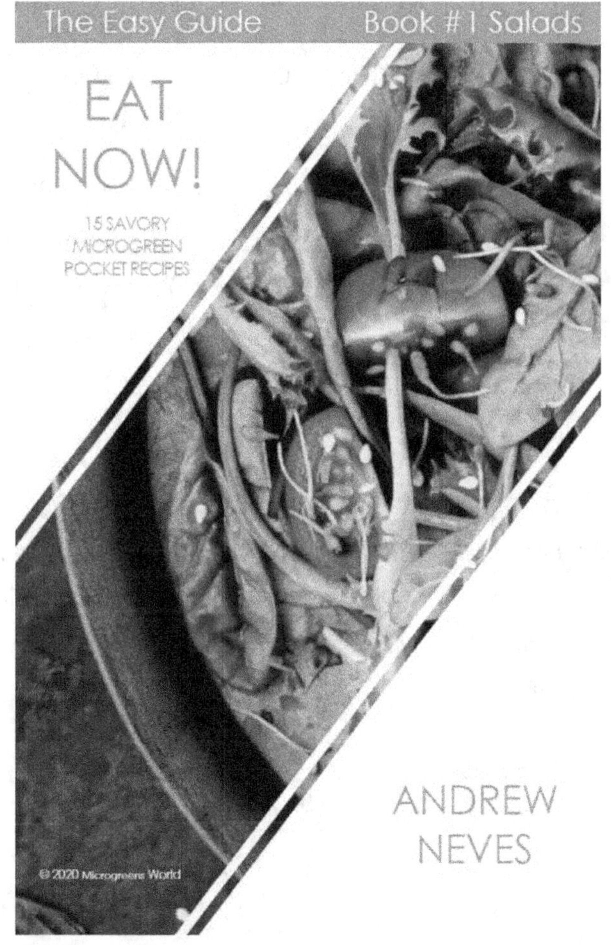

If you like **FREE**, then <u>**CLICK HERE FOR YOUR FREE BOOK**</u>

ABOUT THE AUTHOR

Hi, I'm Andrew Neves, and this is Microgreens World.
Come with me on a journey, as we experiment and
taste and learn together about the latest on
microgreens – Nutrition | Research | Trends

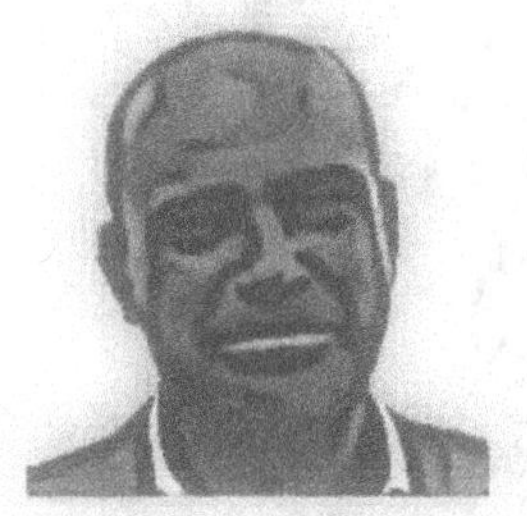

Our family dinners start with
vegetables, grain, and whatever
meat you want. Every meal must
have something "green" on it,
and it's not Jell-O, LOL!

In 2019 a friend introduced my
wife and me to microgreens. They were flavorful
and tasty on our evening meal. Then we started
hanging out at some of the better restaurants in the
city. Everyone, it seemed, was talking about these
microgreens.

Read more here:
https://microgreensworld.com/about/